D1760331

Understanding
Incontinence

WITHDRAWN

Health Library
Clinical Education Centre
ST4 6QG

The Library
College of Nursing and Midwifery
City General Hospital
Stoke on Trent ST4 6QG

RC 921.J5
.M2

Understanding Incontinence

A GUIDE TO THE NATURE
AND MANAGEMENT OF A
VERY COMMON COMPLAINT

Dorothy Mandelstam MCSP DipSocSc

With illustrations by Brenda Naylor

The Library
College of Nursing and Midwifery
City General Hospital
Stoke on Trent ST4 6QG

Published for the Disabled Living Foundation by

CHAPMAN AND HALL

20111.

Published by Heinemann Health Books in 1977
under the title *Incontinence: A guide to the
understanding and management of a very common
complaint*

This revised edition published in 1989 by
Chapman and Hall Ltd
11 New Fetter Lane, London EC4P 4EE

© 1989 Disabled Living Foundation,
380–384 Harrow Road, London W9 2HU

Typeset in 11/12pt Palatino by
Acorn Bookwork, Salisbury, Wilts
Printed in Great Britain by
Mackay's of Chatham PLC
Chatham, Kent

ISBN 0 412 33310 4

This paperback edition is sold subject to the condition that it
shall not, by way of trade or otherwise, be lent, resold, hired
out, or otherwise circulated without the publisher's
prior consent in any form of binding or cover other than that
in which it is published and without a similar
condition including this condition being imposed on the
subsequent purchaser.

All rights reserved. No part of this book may be reprinted or
reproduced, or utilized in any form or by any electronic,
mechanical or other means, now known or hereafter
invented, including photocopying and recording, or in any
information storage and retrieval system, without
permission in writing from the publisher.

British Library Cataloguing in Publication Data

Mandelstam, Dorothy
    Understanding incontinence.
    1. Man. Incontinence.
    I. Title
    616.6'3

    ISBN 0–412–33310–4

Contents

Acknowledgements   vii

Preface   ix

Foreword   xi

Introduction   xiii

1   Focus on incontinence   1

2   Urinary incontinence   5

3   Faecal (bowel) incontinence   14

4   Management of incontinence   18

5   Aids to continence and hygiene   31

6   Protective equipment   46

7   Services available   57

   Appendices:

   A   Suppliers of protective equipment and aids to continence   61

   B   Useful addresses   64

   C   Further reading   69

   Glossary   73

   Index   77

Acknowledgements

In producing this book I am grateful to Lady Hamilton who saw the need for a text of this kind and asked me to write it many years ago. It was first published in 1977 under the title *Incontinence: A guide to the understanding and management of a very common complaint*.

My thanks are also due to Diana de Deney, editor of Disabled Living Foundation publications, and to Brenda Naylor for her sympathetic illustrations.

I am also indebted to many colleagues, especially to Dr M Stewart with whom I worked at Edgware General Hospital.

The Library
College of Nursing and Midwifery
City General Hospital
Stoke on Trent ST4 6QG

Preface

In this small book I have attempted to look at and discuss the subject of incontinence in the hope that the reader will be able to understand the problem and know what kind of help to seek.

Since an earlier version of the book was published in 1977 (under the title of *Incontinence: A guide to the understanding and management of a very common complaint*) there has been an increase in the services for the incontinent person. There are more doctors and more continence advisers who have special expertise. Details of specialist clinics and nurses can be obtained from the Incontinence Advisory Service of the Disabled Living Foundation (DLF).

However, incontinence is still a taboo subject. Any article about the subject in a magazine or television programme inevitably brings hundreds of enquiries from people who are either too embarrassed to seek help or who do not know where to find it.

There are two professional organizations which concentrate on incontinence. The International Continence Society for the most part has a medical membership, and the Association of Continence Advisers has mainly nursing members, but both organizations include other professionals working in this field. Each sets out to study and improve the methods of treating and managing incontinence.

There is a great variety of equipment available and, with increasing information about its use, this aspect of management could be much improved. Education is needed, both for the health service worker and for members of the public. Many manufacturers are actively involved in efforts to encourage the informed use of their products.

Incontinence is costly in terms of human misery. It affects family relationships and can determine where a person lives. The incontinent person may be unwelcome and he or she is acutely aware of this. It is hoped that this book will encourage them to seek help and so improve their situation.

Dorothy Mandelstam MCSP, Dip SocSc

The Library
College of Nursing and Midwifery
City General Hospital
Stoke on Trent ST4 6QG

Foreword

The manuscript of *Incontinence: A guide to the understanding and management of a very common complaint* by Dorothy Mandelstam, MCSP, DipSocSc, was completed in 1976 and the book published in 1977. Although much has changed since that date, much remains unchanged. The changes, however, demanded that the book be updated. This new book is published under a different title – *Understanding Incontinence*.

Incontinence remains a source of shame and distress to the sufferer, and a source of unceasing embarrassment and drudgery to carers. It is a disability of enormous prevalence, and yet is still difficult to mention. However, largely due to publicity on television and radio, and not because it has been mentioned in the printed media (other than the professional press), it is perhaps true to say that the subject is less shunned than it once was.

The DLF has run an Incontinence Advisory Service since 1974, and we know from the people who approach us for help how much still remains to be done. The Incontinence Advisory Service is partially supported by the DHSS, and the DLF Trustees would like to take this opportunity of thanking the Department for the help which it gives. The Service has steadily developed to meet the needs of those professionally concerned and of the public for information and advice. For professional people who care it offers advice on how incontinence can best be helped.

The formation of the Association of Continence Advisers in 1981 has brought about a great improvement. Note that it is an Association of *Continence* Advisers and not of *Incontinence* Advisers, indicating a positive effort to return to continence rather than a reliance on the passive handling of a destructive disability. Dorothy Mandelstam pioneered the Association of Continence Advisers and has been Chairman since its inception. At the time of writing it has 800 members widely distributed throughout the country. Many of them operate as the information resource for their individual area, so that in many parts of the UK there is now a knowledgeable professional person to whom incontinent people and their families can turn for help, and from whom professionals can seek advice. The Association's office is located at the DLF in London.

Dorothy Mandelstam has been the DLF's Incontinence Adviser since 1974. In the last 14 years she has dealt with every kind of enquiry, some of them very complex, to which the disability can give rise. During that time she has also advised and treated individual incontinent patients through her work at the Edgware General Hospital and the Royal Free Hospital. Her very practical book is based on immense experience, and a truly down-to-earth approach, both to the problems and to the positive steps for the return of continence. The DLF Trustees remain deeply grateful to Dorothy Mandelstam for her important work in an almost hidden area of disability. The Trustees also once more thank Mrs Brenda Naylor, the sympathetic illustrator of the book.

Such is the influence of television, radio and the press that it is the media which could now offer the incontinent person the greatest help. If incontinence was mentioned more frequently, the public would gradually begin to accept that it is a permissible subject for discussion and sufferers would find it easier to approach their doctors and others for advice. It is indeed strange that all sorts of sexual practices may be mentioned in detail, but that this widespread disability is not.

Meanwhile, the DLF continues to develop the Incontinence Advisory Service and to publish reference and briefing material for those affected and those who care for them, including those who care for them professionally. It is our hope that this new updated book may be truly useful to a great many people.

W. M. Hamilton CBE, MA
Chairman, Disabled Living Foundation

Introduction

Incontinence is a problem which far too many people have to put up with. There are many reasons for this, partly shame and an unwillingness to reveal that it is present, partly a feeling of hopelessness that nothing can be done, and sometimes because doctors and nurses seem particularly negative in their approach, and this often stems from a lack of knowledge on their part. So much has been discovered about incontinence during the last ten to twenty years that it is only now that medical and nursing schools are beginning to teach their students about its implications. Yet incontinence is a symptom and just as with any other symptom (for instance pain, fever, vomiting or weakness) it needs to be approached with a full history and examination and quite often additional tests must be done to discover its cause. It is only once the cause has been discovered that treatment can be effective.

Dorothy Mandelstam's book has proved to be important in helping to dispel this ignorance, and a demand for this updated version confirms its effectiveness in this regard. The book sets out clearly and simply to treat this ignorance. It also presents information about a whole range of appliances, special clothing and so on, which is helpful in the management of incontinence in those cases where it cannot be cured. The importance of first making a diagnosis and considering specific therapy is indicated and, if this is done effectively, then the proportion of patients who will need to use appliances of various types on a long term basis will be relatively small.

This small book is a mine of information and will be of the greatest use not only to incontinent people but also to those who look after them, and in particular doctors and nurses.

J. C. Brocklehurst MD, FRCP
Professor of Geriatric Medicine
University of Manchester

1
Focus on incontinence

During many years' experience as a physiotherapist and social worker I have been involved with incontinence in gynaecological and geriatric care, both in hospitals, residential homes and with people in their own homes. As adviser on this subject to the Disabled Living Foundation and the Royal Free Hospital, London, I have become increasingly aware of the need for a greater understanding of incontinence, and for advice in dealing with it.

The purpose of this book is to try to fill this need. It is not a textbook, but its aim is to show that incontinence in all its varying aspects can be prevented, treated, alleviated or managed with dignity, and that recognizing the problem is the first step towards finding a solution.

What is incontinence? It is a loss of control over the bladder or bowels. How many suffer it and who are they? They are innumerable. There is the unhappy young man who wets his bed, the schoolgirl who has occasional accidents while giggling, the young mother who has had incomplete control since her baby was born and who, when she reaches middle age, will have even less control, and the isolated and housebound elderly person. In addition to these, there are many people who are disabled, either physically or mentally, and those suffering from an acute illness or injury. Incontinence is a symptom that may occur to any of us at any age.

2 Focus on incontinence

It has been estimated that in this country alone there are possibly two million people suffering from incontinence. A number of these, finding no help elsewhere for one reason or another, write to the Disabled Living Foundation. Any publicity such as a mention in a magazine brings in a spate of letters revealing problems which have often existed for years. Is it surprising that incontinence is regarded with dismay? Its consequences are unpleasant and difficult to hide, and it disturbs our senses as well as our feelings about personal privacy. It is natural that people try to conceal it, even though this may make treatment impossible.

Much incontinence could be prevented by a wider dissemination of knowledge, not only about its physical aspects but also its emotional and social implications.

Causes of incontinence can be diagnosed and treated in a variety of ways by the medical profession; as well as the family doctor there are specialists concerned with the subject. Those who have this problem need to understand their own type of incontinence since, as will be explained in later chapters of this book, there are often ways in which they can help themselves either to maintain control or to gain it. Finally, where some degree of incontinence has to be accepted, it can be managed by the use of the right equipment, but for this to be effective the special requirements of each individual need to be considered.

Incontinence is a condition which has been known for centuries but there are few references to it in the literature, medical or otherwise. The Egyptians and the Greeks recorded various treatments – one of the earliest in the Egyptian medical Papyrus Ebers, dates back to 1500 BC. References have also been found to appliances designed to prevent the involuntary passing of urine.

During the past 2000 years in Western Europe incontinence in children has had more attention than that in adults, and details of treatment for them can be found, particularly dating from the 16th century. One of the first English books on the diseases of children, written in 1544 by Thomas Phaer, the father of paediatrics, contained a chapter 'Of Pyssing in the Bed'. Bedwetting has been regarded as a problem in most societies including some primitive communities; many remedies have been tried, including the use and abuse of fear and punishment. Adult problems have not attracted so much attention, except for those in relation to women and childbirth. In 1777 Thomas Leake, a teacher of midwidery, described two devices for the prevention of incontinence, otherwise there is little recorded.

There are several possible reasons for this. Perhaps under the living conditions of the past incontinence did not present a problem: in Europe during the Middle Ages, and even much later, standards of domestic hygiene were very low; the streets were unpaved and accumulations of human as well as animal excrement produced odours which would be found unacceptable today; underclothing did not exist and bedding consisted of disposable straw. Under these conditions, the effects of incontinence would have passed unnoticed.

The development of higher standards of social and domestic hygiene and cleanliness has unfortunately been accompanied by taboos and inhibitions connected with bodily functions. Britain and the United States have fared the worst in this respect, the Americans being even more prudish than ourselves with their emphasis on sterile lavatories and silent flushing systems.

In this atmosphere of secrecy an incontinent person can only feel shame and embarrassment. Freud wrote on his *Introductory Essays on Psychoanalysis* that the child feels no disgust for its own excreta until this is inculcated by the parents. By comparing one culture with another it can be seen that this feeling of embarrassment can be artificially engendered by social attitudes. In Hindu society it is polite to ask a guest about the state of his bowels, while in this country such a remark would be unthinkable. Our embarrassment is shown by the number of words we use to describe the room where these functions are performed: lavatory, water closet, WC, toilet, littlest room, powder room, ladies' room and many others.

Until recently incontinence held little interest for the medical profession. Perhaps its existence was often not divulged to the doctor, as is sometimes still the case today; also it is not lethal in itself and in most cases can be endured. However, attitudes are gradually changing. Incontinence should not be allowed to make people feel social outcasts or to separate them from their families. The admission of an elderly person to hospital because of incontinence could in some cases be avoided by timely advice and help. With the number of elderly in the population increasing there is a great need for preventative action. Yet incontinence is a word which is rarely heard; few people talk about it although the number of articles in magazines and radio and television programmes are gradually increasing. Many more medical people are now actively involved in developing methods of investigation and treatment, but a greater acceptance by society of the widespread existence of incontinence would help both those who have to endure it and those who are attempting to find remedies.

2

Urinary incontinence

Incontinence may be urinary (connected with the bladder) or faecal (connected with the bowels). Urinary incontinence is by far the most common. It may be helpful to describe the workings of the bladder and the way in which control is acquired in early life.

The bladder (Figure 2.1) lies in the pelvis, a bony basin situated at the lower part of the spine. There is no bony wall in part of the front and no bone at the base. The bladder is a thin-walled muscular sac with an outlet tube called the urethra. It is the reservoir for the collection of urine and can be distended to contain 1 pint (0.5 litres) or more of urine. Urine is carried to the bladder from the

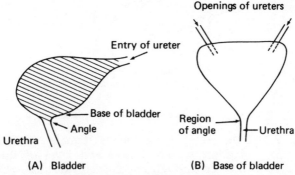

(A) Bladder   (B) Base of bladder

Figure 2.1   (A and B) The bladder.

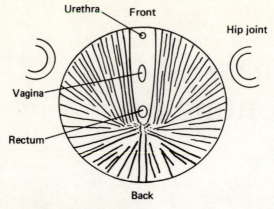

Urethra = urine passage
Vagina = front passage
Rectum = back passage

Figure 2.2 Muscular floor of the pelvis (female), viewed from above.

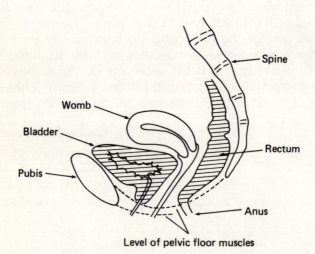

Level of pelvic floor muscles

Figure 2.3 Side view of the pelvis (female), showing the bladder, womb, bowel and level of the pelvic muscles through which their exit tubes pass.

kidneys by two tubes (ureters), the ends of which pass obliquely through the muscular bladder wall and open into the base of the bladder (trigone). The urethra leads out of the front of the base at an angle; this angle functions as a valve keeping the urethra closed except during the process of passing water (micturition).

Like other organs within the pelvis (Figures 2.2 and 2.3) the bladder is supported by a floor consisting of two flat muscles. There is a gap between them at the front through which the exit tubes of the organs pass. The edges of the gap can be brought together by conscious tightening of the muscles, and in so doing stop the passage of urine or faeces. This is helped by a superficial but smaller layer of muscle, which also plays a part in maintaining continence (see exercises, p. 20). Passing water is such an ordinary act that we take it for granted, but in fact it is quite a complicated process.

CONTROL OF THE BLADDER

In an infant before it is trained, the bladder acts automatically. Emptying occurs as soon as the urine within the bladder reaches a certain volume, the accompanying rise in pressure resulting in contractions of the bladder which expel the urine. This is a spontaneous and unconscious act controlled by a centre in the spinal cord. As the small child develops, control from the brain is gradually established (Figure 2.4), making it possible for the voiding of urine to be postponed. With guidance from the mother, the child learns to pass water only in suitable places and also to go at convenient times even in the absence of any urge. This training may take two years or more, and everyone recognizes that children frequently have accidents during this period, for instance when they are totally preoccupied in play.

Some adults, having failed to develop control of the bladder in childhood, continue to wet the bed (adult enuresis).

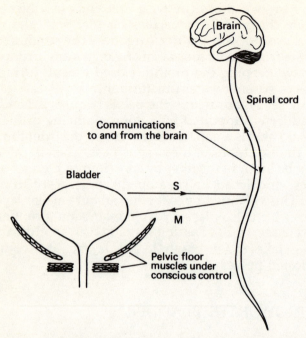

Figure 2.4 Control of the bladder by the brain. Unconscious sensations (S) pass from the bladder to the spinal cord, and unconscious messages (M) pass from the spinal cord to the bladder. Bladder control by the brain becomes established as the child 'grows up'.

Natural variations

Following childhood, complete urinary control is achieved by most people, but individual habits of urination vary greatly. Some pass water more frequently than others. Children, rather than use unpleasant school lavatories, learn to control their bladders until they arrive home, often holding on to a large volume of urine in the process. Some people, indeed most elderly people, need to get up in the night – the chamber pot, now seldom seen, certainly had its uses.

What can go wrong?

There are many different causes of incontinence. These include temporary illness, childbirth, local conditions affecting the bladder or womb (some forms of prolapse), complications of the arteries, and injury or disease of the spinal cord. Incontinence may take various forms, depending on the cause, so it is important to define the nature of the leakage as this can give a clue to the underlying problem.

TYPES OF LEAKAGE

The following will be described:

1. stress incontinence – a small leakage on exertion, e.g. coughing, sneezing;
2. urge incontinence – urgency and frequency leading to a large leakage;
3. overflow incontinence – dribbles or spurts;
4. reflex incontinence – large leakage of urine with no sensation from bladder;
5. nocturnal incontinence – passing of urine during sleep.

Stress incontinence

In this condition urine leaks out during some slight exertion, such as a cough or sneeze, and in some women even when walking or turning in bed. The main reason for this is the overstretching and laxity of the supporting structures around the urethra (bladder neck) and the weakness of the muscles of the pelvic floor. Both the supporting structures and the muscles normally contribute to keeping the urethra closed. This type of incontinence frequently follows childbirth, though women who have not had children can be affected. As long as the leakage is small it does not present a major problem. However, the condition is likely to become more troublesome as the years pass if no action is taken. Unfortunately, many women accept it as an inevitable consequence of childbirth; they do not mention it to the doctor and it is often not recognized at post-natal examinations. This form of incontinence is estimated to affect 20% of all women at some period in their lives. Nowadays most women are taught pelvic floor exercises after having a baby, and these, if practised conscientiously at the time, do much to prevent stress incontinence developing; for this reason effective post-natal teaching is of paramount importance.

Urge incontinence

Urgency is a wish to pass water at once, which if not satisfied may lead to incontinence. It is often accompanied by the need to pass water frequently (increased frequency).

Precipitancy is similar to urgency, except that there is no warning time; as soon as the desire to pass water is felt, urine pours out.

Urgency and frequency are symptoms of the irritability of the muscle of the bladder and can be caused by a urinary infection (cystitis) or other irritation of the lining of the bladder. The desire to pass urine frequently may also be due to habit (p. 21).

These symptoms, together with precipitancy, can also develop gradually as result of decreasing control of the bladder from the brain centre. They may follow an injury to the brain, a stroke or disease of the blood vessels in the brain. They may also be caused by pressure around the outlet of the bladder, as in enlargement of the prostate gland in men.

Overflow incontinence – dribbling

This term is used when urine flows in drops or a trickling stream causing constant dampness. There are many causes. One of the commonest is severe constipation. The hardened bowel motion presses on the bladder tube (urethra) preventing the bladder from emptying naturally.

The bladder continues to be filled with urine, and as it is unable to empty itself small amounts of urine may constantly dribble away.

It can also be associated with enlargement of the prostate gland in men. The gland is situated around the upper part of the urethra and may cause complete or partial obstruction of the flow of urine from the bladder. Similarly, fibroids in the womb may have the same obstructive effect.

Dribbling may also occur as the result of spinal cord diseases affecting the nerves that control the muscles involved in emptying the bladder.

Reflex incontinence

This results in the emptying of the bladder without the individual concerned realizing that it has happened. The nerves conveying messages to and from the bladder may be damaged by illness or an accident.

Nocturnal incontinence

Night-time leakage may occur in sleep, when the desire to pass urine is absent, or is not strong enough to wake the person. Sometimes this may be due to the effect of sleeping tablets.

Others who are woken by the need to pass urine once or twice a night may not be able to reach the lavatory in time and an accident may result (Chapter 5).

OTHER FACTORS

There are emotional and physical factors which, while not connected with urinary function, may result in incontinence.

Emotional factors

Emotion can affect the action of the bladder. It is quite common to feel the desire to pass water when under some temporary strain, for example before an important interview, or when frightened. In an adult an emotional shock such as bereavement may produce an episode of incontinence.

Emotional wellbeing plays a part in the complicated mechanism of continence. If an elderly person is leading a lonely life, hopelessness and apathy may lead to inactivity, immobility and the occurrence of 'accidents'. Forgetfulness and mild confusion can also upset normal habits. Admission to a strange environment, like a hospital, and dependence on others for bodily needs may cause unhappiness and have a similar effect. Some doctors think that severe distress can in itself be a cause of the breakdown of the patterns of a lifetime, resulting in an inability to perform bodily functions in the accustomed places, with consequent wetting and soiling. This behaviour is not deliberate, and requires carers to be patient and understanding. On the other hand, someone who has been incontinent during a period of difficulty or loneliness at home may regain control in hospital.

A word is needed about the emotional effects of incontinence on the sufferer. These can be devastating and lead to bizarre behaviour. Some people try pathetically to conceal wet or soiled pads or clothing in an attempt to deny the problem. This may seem a 'dirty' habit but it is in fact a call for help.

Physical disabilities

Arthritis may result in difficult and slow walking; if there is an urgent need to urinate and the toilet is not reached in time, incontinence will follow. Any disability of the hands and arms and, in women, inability to bend at the hips, may aggravate the situation. These factors have to be taken into account when planning the management of incontinence (Chapters 4 and 5).

Medicines

If confusion and drowsiness are produced by sedatives or tranquillizers incontinence may result. Diuretics (water pills) which cause the kidneys to produce more urine may give rise to urgency and frequency.

The Library
College of Nursing and Midwifery
City General Hospital
Stoke on Trent ST4 6QG

3

Faecal (bowel) incontinence

The process of digestion and absorption is constantly
going on and the intestines are continuously propelling
their contents onward toward the rectum (the last part of
the bowel) for the final discharge of any unabsorbed
residue. For most of the time the rectum is not loaded
(Figure 3.1).

Following some habitual stimulus the contents of the
large bowel are passed along into the rectum which now
becomes distended with faeces. When a certain degree of
distension is reached, the rectum as a whole starts to
contract and empty itself. Passage of a motion can be
voluntarily prevented or controlled by the contraction of
the pelvic floor muscles together with the ring-like muscle
around the external opening of the bowel (anus). Contraction of these muscles allows the rectum to dilate and retain
faeces for varying lengths of time.

The motion when passed should be soft, well-formed
and easy to pass, otherwise undue strain is put on the
pelvic muscles. Constipation produced by postponing the
passing of stool will increase the strain.

Natural variations

While a regular daily bowel action may be desirable, there
is individual variation. A survey has shown that while the

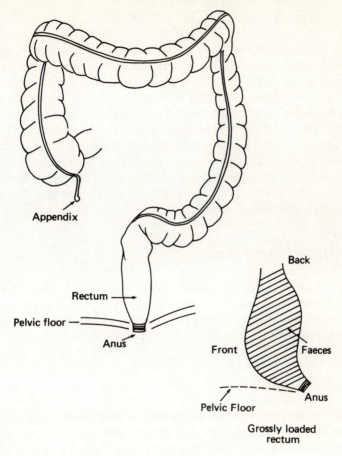

Figure 3.1 The large bowel, rectum and anus.

normal habit for some may be three times a day, for others it may be three times a week. It is therefore important to know an individual's normal habit, and the conditions necessary to maintain it, such as time of day when a motion is passed, pattern of exercise, diet, drinking habits, etc. It is common knowledge that holidays or other environmental changes can upset such a routine; in fact any emotional upset or change of lifestyle may alter it.

CAUSES OF FAECAL INCONTINENCE

The most common form of faecal incontinence is some-times known as overflow diarrhoea. It is caused by a long standing accumulation of bowel matter in the rectum (severe constipation). The motion cannot be passed nor-mally and a liquid that looks like diarrhoea seeps past the bowel matter from higher up the bowel. As mentioned on p. 10 severe constipation also causes urinary incontinence.

Faecal incontinence can also be caused by damage to the anal sphincter (back passage) during childbirth or surgery, or if sphincteric control is lost due to coma, illness, nervous disease or spinal injury.

DOUBLE INCONTINENCE

This term is used to describe a condition of both urinary and faecal incontinence existing together. Double inconti-nence is frequently caused by severe constipation (faecal impaction).

MANAGEMENT

The results of faecal incontinence may be more unpleasant than those of urinary incontinence. Attention to possible causes and positive management may help to prevent it, or at least make control more possible.

Overflow diarrhoea – due to constipation can be treated, and should be preventable.

PREVENTION

Bowel activity can be a source of worry to many people. In order to alleviate these worries and prevent constipation, and worse still, faecal incontinence, the following points need to be considered:

1. how regular is the normal bowel habit? As this varies with individuals it is useful to keep a record of the pattern. How often is a motion passed; is it soft and well-formed, or is there pain and discomfort when it is passed?
2. when were the bowels last opened?
3. are the bowels stimulated by any particular event, such as drinking a glass of hot water first thing in the morning or last thing at night?
4. are laxatives taken regularly? Or any drugs which might have a constipating effect?
5. drinks should not be reduced, as this may affect the bowel habits.
6. a good diet, with wholemeal bread, cereals, fresh fruit and vegetables, maintain regular bowel activity. Sometimes bran, or other preparations like Fybogel or Isogel (available from any chemist), are needed to add bulk to the diet. These are different from laxatives, which are not meant to be used on a long term basis.

PERSISTENT INCONTINENCE

If this occurs it may be due to a number of different causes and advice from a doctor is essential.

If protection is needed, pads with a plastic backing would be suitable (p. 51).

4
Management of incontinence

IMPORTANCE OF ATTITUDE

We are accustomed to being able to manage those bodily functions which are under our voluntary control and it is distressing when that control is lost. Incontinence is therefore an embarrassing subject and it is often necessary to dispel the emotion-charged atmosphere which accompanies the condition. In the first place a sympathetic approach on the part of the relative, nurse or attendant is essential to help the affected person overcome any feelings of shame. This is not easy, as in our civilized society the waste products of the body (excreta) tend to be regarded as unpleasant or even disgusting. Incontinence may arouse feelings of hostility in those who have to care for the incontinent person, possibly because of the apparent hopelessness of ever resolving or improving the condition. Professional help and advice, and moral support for the relative, can transform this situation and consequently improve relationships. A matter-of-fact attitude is reassuring since the incontinent person may be anxious not only about soiling himself or herself but about giving trouble to others as a result. Once the confidence of the sufferer is gained the aim of further management is to enable him or her to cope with the problem and become as independent as possible.

URINARY INCONTINENCE

It is important first to determine the nature of the incontinence. Initially a visit to the family doctor is essential. It will help him or her if the sufferer is able to answer the following questions:

1. how long have you been troubled this way?
2. did it start suddenly or gradually? Was it associated with any particular event?
3. do you have a small leakage of urine on slight exertion, such as coughing, sneezing, laughing, or even turning over in bed (stress incontinence)? Or is the leakage on exertion considerable (unstable bladder plus stress incontinence)?
4. do you feel the need to pass urine more frequently than usual during the day? How often? And also at night? How often? Are you drinking more fluid than usual?
5. do you have a feeling of urgency? How much warning time do you get?
6. do you ever have an 'accident' (urge incontinence)?
7. do you wet yourself without being aware of passing urine? Is the leakage a little or a lot (retention with overflow incontinence; reflex emptying)?

After discussion, the family doctor may wish to refer a patient to a specialist in a centre for further investigation. There are a number of incontinence/urodynamic clinics in the UK where medical and nursing staff have a particular concern for incontinence problems as well as expertise in new methods of assessment and management.

Stress incontinence

This can be treated by re-education of muscles or by surgery or both.

Exercises

In many women this type of leakage which occurs on coughing, laughing, sneezing or lifting, can be corrected by exercising the pelvic floor muscles (which support the bladder), providing practice is persistent and carried out over a period of time.

The following exercises should achieve results:

1. sit, stand or lie and, without tensing the muscles of your legs, buttocks or abdomen, tighten the ring of muscles around the anus by imagining that you are trying to control the passing of a stool. This will help you identify the back part of the pelvic floor;
2. when you are passing urine, try to stop the flow, then restart it. Do this once a day when you empty your bladder. Gradually you will become aware of the front muscles of the pelvic floor;
3. working them back to front, tighten the pelvic floor muscles while counting to four slowly, then release them. Do this four times every hour, for the next three months. You can do this exercise anywhere – sitting or standing, while watching television or waiting for a bus. There is no need to interrupt your normal daily activity.

After practising for two to three weeks, you will feel the closure of the back and front passages, and a drawing up of the pelvic floor in front.

Do these exercises without tightening the abdominal, thigh or buttock muscles or crossing your legs, otherwise you may not be working the right internal muscles. The movement is distinct and separate from the others, and women can check this, while in the bath or shower, by placing one finger inside the birth passage and contracting the pelvic floor muscles.

Following childbirth some women are aware of diminished sensation during intercourse. Others leak urine during intercourse which can be embarrassing. Both are due to the stretching of structures around the vagina. The exercises just described will help to improve both problems.

Surgery
Other women whose pelvic muscles and surrounding structures are considerably weakened may need surgery.

There are several operations which can be performed to tighten up the structures under the bladder (bladder neck and urethra) either through the vagina (birth passage) or through the abdomen. The method used will depend on a number of individual factors, which the doctor will discuss with the patient.

The vaginal repair requires five to seven days in hospital, and the abdominal methods about two weeks. A period of convalescence of a few weeks to three months may follow, during which time it is best to avoid lifting and abdominal exertion. It is advisable to wait for six weeks before resuming sexual intercourse to allow for full healing.

Urge incontinence – urgency, frequency

If urgency and frequency occur suddenly, it may be due to an infection or some other cause of irritation in the bladder, and a doctor should be consulted.

Bladder training
If the onset has been gradual it may be due to other causes and the following suggestions may be tried. Sometimes a habit of frequent emptying develops, especially if there is anxiety about having a bladder accident. A plan to retrain the bladder may help:

1. note on a piece of paper when urine is passed, and how much fluid is drunk during the day;
2. The next day, each time the need to pass urine is felt, an attempt should be made to hold on for five minutes longer;
3. if the above is difficult, sitting on the edge of a hard chair and pulling up the pelvic muscles (see p. 20) will help to control the urge to pass water;
4. holding on for longer each day should be continued each time the desire to pass urine is felt. This should

be gradual, starting from 5 minutes and working up to 60 minutes waiting time, and even longer. In this way there should be a return to a normal pattern of passing water five to six times a day. This may take several weeks.

Physical difficulties

Some elderly people who have urgency may find that the lavatory is too far away to be reached in time, especially if walking is slow. To prevent accidents, a substitute lavatory could be considered. A commode, bedpan or urinal would help solve the problem, especially at night (Chapter 5).

Overflow incontinence

Constipation

If overflow incontinence is due to constipation the cause can easily be confirmed by the doctor or nurse, by an examination through the back passage. It can be corrected by the use of an enema, suppository, or, if necessary, by manual evacuation. Thereafter, a suitable regime of diet and medicine (sometimes) needs to be followed to ensure a regular bowel action, and the incontinence should not return. Advice may be needed to work out the most suitable regime. For further details see Chapter 3 on faecal incontinence.

The advice of the family doctor, however, is essential as there are other causes of overflow incontinence and surgical or medical care may be required.

Prostate gland

If this gland has become enlarged leading to overflow incontinence, surgery may be required. This is a common operation and is usually performed through the bladder tube (transurethral resection) and is done under a general anaesthetic. It takes about one hour. The length of stay in hospital is about one week, and convalescence three to four weeks. During this time the passing of water may at first be frequent and somewhat uncomfortable and a little blood may be passed. Gradually the bladder returns to normal but it is advisable to avoid constipation, heavy lifting and to abstain from sexual activity for four to six weeks. If there is a slight leakage of urine during this time it helps to retrain the bladder by holding on to the urine for longer periods using the pelvic muscles at the outlet (see p. 20).

Reflex incontinence

As there is no awareness of the need to pass urine, a routine can sometimes be imposed on the bladder. Urine should be passed at regular intervals, for instance every two hours. In this way the bladder learns to respond, emptying itself into a lavatory and for the most part dryness is achieved. It may be necessary to wear a pad as an extra protection.

The use of intermittent self-catheterization (see spinal injury, p. 28) may be another solution. This technique can only be applied after consultation with a doctor. Advice and teaching of the method can be obtained at an incontinence clinic, or from a continence nurse adviser. The method has been used for some time for people who have suffered spinal injuries. It is now being used more widely for others who have a similar type of incontinence caused by other conditions.

Long term catheterization may also be used.

LONG TERM CATHETERIZATION

The insertion of a catheter may be the answer to a difficult and uncontrollable form of incontinence. A small tube is placed through the urethra into the bladder and the urine is drained into a bag. The doctor will decide if this is a suitable method to be used.

If this long term catheterization is used the catheter will need to be changed about every six weeks to three months. The district nurse will change the catheter and give advice about its management, but these are some useful suggestions:

1. drink freely;
2. avoid constipation;
3. avoid kinking the tube, and keep the bag below the exit of the tube;
4. when a day bag is changed for a night bag (usually larger) it should be washed out with warm water and a mild detergent. The bag will last for about one week;
5. the bag can be concealed on the leg, either on the thigh or calf, either by straps, or held in a special holder (see below, also pp 48–50).

Sex and a catheter

If a catheter is inserted it is not easy to have sex with it in place. There may be a reluctance to talk about this situation but it is worthwhile discussing it with the doctor or nurse as there may be alternative methods.

In some circumstances a catheter can be inserted through the abdomen (suprapubic catheter) instead of through the bladder outlet, thus making intercourse easier. Alternatively, it may be possible to teach either partner to remove the catheter before, and reinsert it after, sex.

Again, a change of position during sex from the back to the side may make intercourse more comfortable for a woman. These matters should be discussed with the doctor to decide which measures would be most suitable. Advice may also be sought from SPOD who supply information on disability and sex (see Appendix B).

SEX AND INCONTINENCE

The bladder exit and the sex organs are close together, and for some people any mention of either is embarrassing. However, if there are incontinence problems it is worthwhile seeking advice.

Many women with stress incontinence leak during

sexual intercourse. Strengthening the pelvic muscles around the bladder outlet can improve this, and incidentally these exercises as already mentioned can improve sexual sensation if it has been diminished because of the stretching of tissues and muscles.

Some women empty the contents of the bladder during an orgasm. If certain practical steps are taken the embarrassment can be lessened; make sure the bladder is emptied before sex and protect the bed with a towel under the buttocks.

Practical measures are even more important if one of the partners wets the bed during sleep. This is often an upsetting situation for both, and may lead to difficulties in the relationship (see next section).

ADULT BEDWETTING (NOCTURNAL ENURESIS)

Wetting the bed during sleep is a problem for many people; it is upsetting and causes embarrassment particularly when marriage or the taking of a partner is contemplated. Some people feel it is a childish habit which they have never outgrown, and are therefore reluctant to admit it.

While there is often no obvious physical or mental cause of bedwetting advice should still be sought. There are now specialist centres (urodynamic or incontinence clinics) where these problems can be investigated and practical advice given. Find out from the doctor where the nearest clinic is, or the name of a specialist continence nurse adviser.

Treatment may include the use of drugs, or the use of an enuresis alarm. The alarm or bell and buzzer system is placed on the bed and gives out signals when urine is passed. Signals wake the sleeper who can then empty the bladder. If this system is continued over a number of weeks the person will, eventually, either wake up naturally to empty the bladder or will be able to hold on until the morning. This method has proved very succesful in children, and is equally suitable for adults. It does however require proper use and should be tried over a period of up to three months. Professional advice can be obtained from a nurse adviser. For further reading see Appendix C. Other simple measures may help:

1. drinks – try restricting these at night, especially before sleep. Tea, coffee and alcohol (especially large quantities of beer) can cause the bedwetting or make it worse;
2. charts – keep a record of when the wetting occurs. Some nights may be dry and others wet, so it may be possible to pinpoint the relevant cause;
3. bladder training – it can be helpful to train the bladder in the daytime so that its capacity for holding on to larger quantities of urine is increased. This is done by drinking more and passing urine less frequently (see bladder training on p. 21); with a larger capacity bladder it may be possible to remain dry during the night.

STROKE

Incontinence frequently accompanies the early phase of a stroke, but is not necessarily lasting. Certain mechanical difficulties can arise, however, and these may lead to accidents, but if they are understood, help can be given so that continence is maintained.

First, it is as well to remember that while the patient may not be able to speak clearly or express himself or herself he or she is usually very much aware of what is going on, and particularly concerned about bladder and bowel control. Activity needs to be directed to restoring independence in this respect, bearing in mind the following points:

1. as one side of the body tends to be affected it is more difficult to manage in the lavatory, or to handle a bottle or urinal, using only one hand. A technique worked out with the help of a relative or therapist will not only solve the practical problem but will also help to restore confidence. The right kind of clothing

The Library
College of Nursing and Midwifery
City General Hospital
Stoke on Trent ST4 6QG

(see Chapter 5) can contribute greatly to ease of management.

2. there may be an added difficulty if the patient, when given the bottle, does not know what to do with it. Sometimes recognition of an object either by sight or touch is lost, but if he or she is shown repeatedly how to use it the action will soon be re-learned.
3. where loss of speech makes communication about bodily needs difficult, a system needs to be worked out – perhaps the ringing of a hand-bell when the need to urinate is felt.

It is not possible to know what degree of function can be restored in any particular individual, but every effort should be made to encourage independence especially in relation to bladder and bowel activity. Dependence on others for these needs is demoralizing, but with help and the retraining of certain actions there will usually be a definite improvement.

MANAGEMENT OF SOME SPECIAL CONDITIONS

In a few rare conditions, where incontinence cannot be controlled in any other way, surgical treatment may be required. This may be in the form of a urinary diversion whereby the urine, instead of flowing into the bladder, is diverted to an artificial opening (stoma) in the wall of the abdomen and is collected in a bag, or the ureters are transplanted into the bowel to drain through the rectum.

In some patients where there is loss of control of the nerves supplying the bladder (e.g. spinal injury) an electronic stimulator can be implanted into the lower part of the spine. This can then activate the bladder and empty it. This is a new technique and so far has only been used in relatively small numbers of patients. Another new technical achievement is the implantation of an artificial urinary sphincter. It requires a special surgical technique but can be managed fairly simply by the patient. It is controlled by a pump of which a part is inserted into the genital area. This can then be squeezed by the patient when needing to void urine. At other times continence is maintained. This technique is not widespread and is applied only to selected patients.

SPINAL INJURIES

In many people with spinal injuries the bladder can be retrained, and this training is already available at certain specialist centres. (Information can be obtained from the Spinal Injuries Association – see Appendix B.)

Where bladder sensation is lost it may be possible to stimulate reflex emptying at regular intervals by tapping, kneading or stroking the lower abdomen. Where the bladder is incapable of muscular contractions hand pressure can be used to help emptying.

An alternative method is the use of intermittent self catheterization. The patient is taught how to insert a small soft tube (catheter) through the urethral passage into the bladder to drain away urine, after which it is withdrawn. This is repeated at suitable intervals. This method is gaining more widespread use in adults and children.

For others with uncontrollable urinary incontinence there are appliances which can be fitted to the body; the advice of a surgical appliance expert or continence adviser is required to ensure fit and comfort. There are no devices for women but pads and pants can offer protection (see Chapter 6).

Bowel control

For those with no sensation in the anal region due to injury of the spinal nerves, it is possible to establish a bowel rhythm. This involves inducing a state of mild constipation and stimulating bowel activity at planned times. This can be effected by dietary control, but suppositories and manual removal of stools may be required. This routine should be decided upon in conjunction with professional advisers.

MULTIPLE SCLEROSIS (DISSEMINATED SCLEROSIS)

In this condition there are a number of symptoms, but one of the most awkward to cope with is incontinence. By the very nature of the disease, accompanying urinary symptoms are diverse. Even the name 'multiple' reflects this. Urgency, increased frequency, and precipitancy may occur, lasting perhaps a few weeks, or months or years. In some patients acute retention of urine may be an initial problem, as the sensation of the bladder being full is impaired. The raised pressure in the distended bladder may force small amounts of urine out at intervals causing dribbling (overflow incontinence). Loss of tone in the sphincter muscles may also lead to lack of control.

A useful, practical and informative leaflet has been produced by the Multiple Sclerosis Society. This can be obtained free of charge (see Appendix B).

GOING INTO HOSPITAL

If you are admitted to hospital for any reason, the following suggestions may be helpful:

1. be sure to tell the nurse in charge about your individual personal needs – for example how often you need to pass water, and whether you require a commode by the bed. In some hospitals these are provided, and if you need to go often and very quickly, especially at night, try and obtain one;
2. hospital wards are frequently large and the lavatories may be some distance away. Find out immediately where they are, and whether you can walk there; if you walk slowly, be sure to allow yourself plenty of time;
3. if you have to use a bedpan, do not be shy about asking for it. The nurse will not know your personal needs unless you tell him or her. Using a bedpan may be a little strange at first;
4. most hospitals nowadays have beds of adjustable

height – do not be afraid to say if your bed is too high or too low for you to be able to get in and out comfortably and without help;

5. there may be set times for 'toilet rounds' in your ward, but your bladder may need to be emptied more frequently. Explain this to the nurse in charge;

6. even if you are incontinent at times make sure you satisfy your thirst;

7. it takes some time to settle down in hospital, and your bowel habits may alter as they tend to do on holiday. Try if possible to keep to the same routine as when you are at home, and do not be afraid of letting the nursing staff know what it is – not everyone has a daily bowel action, and 'normal' can mean anything from three times a day to three times a week.

5

Aids to continence and hygiene

There are a number of items of equipment which can be of great use in the management of incontinence, especially if disability makes movement slow and difficult. The addresses of suppliers of special equipment are given in Appendix A.

URINALS

A urinal is a receptacle into which urine can be passed, and as it can be kept nearby it is particularly useful for someone with urgency and very little warning time; it is also useful for someone who cannot move easily.

Male urinals

A conventional male urinal is commonly known as a bottle (Figure 5.1). There are many different makes, some in lightweight plastic (polypropylene), and others in glass or stainless steel. A bottle can be fitted with a non-spill adaptor to prevent spilling in the bed or chair (Thackraycare). There is also a disposable plastic collector with a built-in non-returnable valve (Figure 5.2). These pack flat and are sold in boxes of ten, and would be very useful when travelling or on holiday (Simcare).

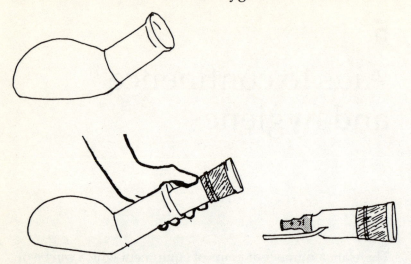

Figure 5.1 Male urinal (bottle) and non-spill adaptors.

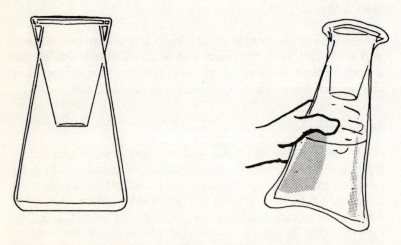

Figure 5.2 Disposable plastic collector with built-in non-returnable valve.

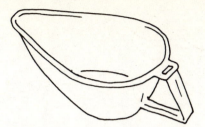

Figure 5.3 St Peter's Boat.

Female urinals

Apart from the familiar type of bedpan used in hospital by both men and women there are urinals and bedpans especially designed for women.

St Peter's Boat (Figure 5.3) is a pointed dish with handle which can be slipped easily between the legs and can be used while standing or sitting (Henleys Medical Supplies Ltd).

Another type is a small shallow dish with an inward-curving, splash-proof rim and a capped hollow handle through which it can be emptied (Figure 5.4). This dish can be slipped under the buttocks without having to raise the hips, and is small enough to manage with one hand (Suba-Seal Urinal, Freeman William and Co. Ltd; Boots; John Bell and Croydon Ltd).

The swan-type urinal (Figure 5.5) is similar to the male bottle, but with a wider neck; it is specially shaped to be held close to the body (Freeman William and Co. Ltd).

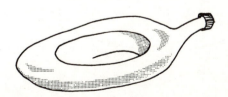

Figure 5.4 Female urinal with splash-proof rim.

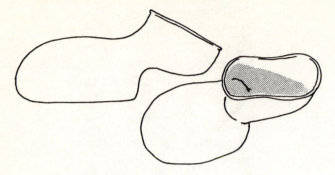

Figure 5.5 Swan-type urinal.

A fracture bedpan (Figure 5.6) is wedge-shaped and designed to be slipped under the body without raising the pelvis. It can be used in a semi-recumbent position (Freeman William and Co. Ltd).

A device of particular use when travelling can be made at home from a soft plastic funnel with a short length of flexible tubing attached; this can empty into a hot water bottle (which can be closed and emptied unobtrusively later (Figure 5.7)). The non-spill disposable plastic container already described could also be used for this.

Another type of urinal available, designed by a research

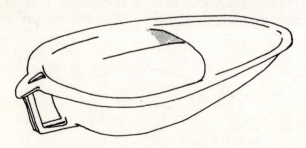

Figure 5.6 Facture bed pan.

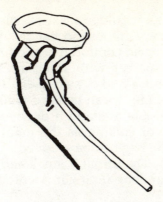

Figure 5.7 Homemade device for use when travelling.

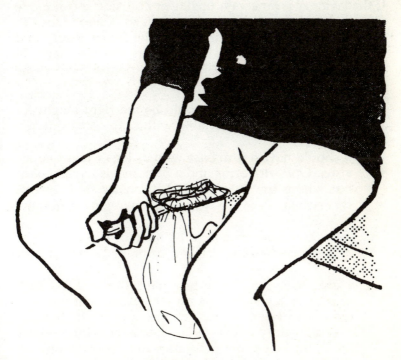

Figure 5.8 Feminal.

nurse, consists of a moulded plastic section, contoured to fit the female body, with a short handle in front by means of which it can be held comfortably and firmly in position. A disposable plastic bag with an elasticated top fits over the rim of the device and is suspended from it to collect the urine (Figure 5.8). It can be used while sitting, standing, and it is possible to stand it down quite safely after use without risk of spilling as the moulded section has straight sides. The bag can be emptied, disposed of, or if necessary reused. The urinal is small and light and could be carried in a handbag (Franklin Medical Ltd).

COMMODES

If the lavatory is far away, upstairs or outside, a commode or a chemical closet can be used instead. Commodes can either be kept in the bedroom or the living room, and some are designed to look like ordinary fireside chairs. In choosing a commode, the following points need to be taken into account:

1. it is important that it should be the right height for the user to sit comfortably with both feet firmly on the floor;
2. it should have a firm base with its legs wider than its arms. One with arms and a back rest is usually best, but where the user needs to transfer from bed or wheelchair there are types with swinging or removable arms;
3. if the commode needs to be moved, it should have castors or wheels which can be braked when it is in use;
4. a sani-chair may be appropriate; this is a lavatory seat set in a chair-frame on wheels, so that the user can be wheeled, or can propel himself or herself, over a lavatory or commode. Before acquiring one of these, the height of the lavatory or commode must be checked to make sure that the sani-chair will go over it.

CUT OUT CUSHIONS

For someone who is unable to move and who spends long periods alone, toiletting may be made easier by a cushion cut to accommodate a female urinal (Figure 5.9), e.g. Suba-Seal (see page 33). There are, however, certain dis-advantages – not everyone finds it easy to sit in the correct position, and some users may find it uncomfortable.

CHEMICAL CLOSETS

A portable lavatory of the kind used when camping or caravanning may sometimes be preferred, as it does not have to be emptied immediately. There are a number of different models, including some with a limited flushing system. Size and stability should be considered as well as capacity; the smaller the model the lighter it will be to

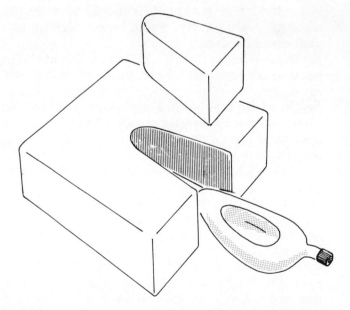

Figure 5.9 Cut-out cushion for use with female urinal.

empty, but for a heavy or disabled user a small closet may need to be placed in a firm-based frame. A chemical commode suitable for domestic use is also available, e.g. Ganmill Ltd.

AIDS IN THE LAVATORY

If the lavatory can be reached there are various ways of making it more comfortable and easier to use. The following suggestions may be helpful:

1. access should be made as easy as possible, and any obstacles removed. If there is insufficient room to manoeuvre inside, perhaps the door could be re-hung so as to open outwards;
2. if the lavatory is cold it can be heated economically by means of a low voltage electrical tubular heater at skirting-board level. This can be left on at all times, but in the interests of safety it should be protected by a guard. Alternatively, a wall heater high up on the wall could be used;
3. for those who have difficulty in bending at the hips, a raised lavatory seat makes sitting down and getting up easier. There are various types which raise the height of the seat by four to six inches (10 to 15 cm). They are placed directly on top of the lavatory pan and some are adjustable to the pan size, as well as adjustable in height (Figure 5.10). Others can be fixed to have a tilt. They are easily removed for normal use;
4. sometimes support is needed when standing or arranging clothing. A grab rail suitably placed on the lavatory wall can be a great help (Figure 5.11), but it is essential that it should be fixed securely enough to take the necessary strain, and at the best angle for the user. An alternative might be a horizontal bar fixed to one or both walls at about waist level.
   Another form of horizontal support consists of a drop-down bar, fixed to the wall behind the lavatory,

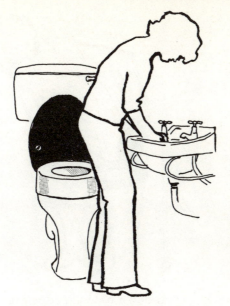

Figure 5.10 Raised lavatory seat.

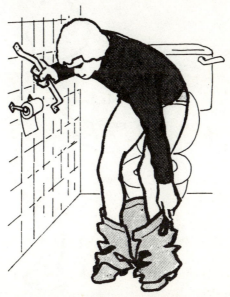

Figure 5.11 Grab rail.

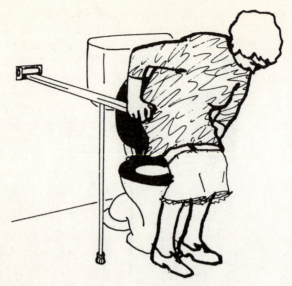

Figure 5.12 Drop-down bar with supporting leg.

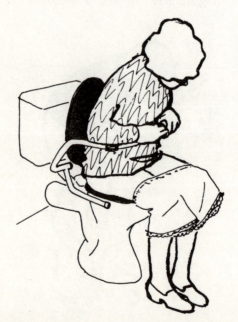

Figure 5.13 Rail designed to close across the front of the user.

with a drop-down, right-angled supporting leg (Figure 5.12); this has the advantage of folding back against the wall when not in use, and so gives access for wheelchair users. There are also chrome rails which are designed to close across the front of the user, to give all round support to the frail or unsteady (Figure 5.13). This support is locked in place through the mounting holes of the lavatory seat, and the enclosing arms swing back out of the way for getting on and off the lavatory;

5. some walking frames are of a design to fit across the lavatory and provide support getting on and off (Figure 5.14);

6. it is important the toilet paper should be placed so that it can be reached without difficulty, especially if there is restricted use of one arm or hand. A box of interleaved paper or paper handkerchief tissues may be easier to manage than a toilet roll. All toilet paper should be soft for maximum efficiency of action.

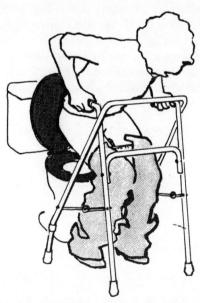

Figure 5.14 Walking frame which fits across the lavatory.

AIDS IN WASHING AND BATHING

1. Cleansing and washing while sitting on the lavatory itself can be made easier by the fitting of a horse-shoe shaped lavatory seat with a front opening (Nicholls & Clark Ltd). A portable bidet (Figure 5.15) is another useful device; this is a shallow plastic bowl which can be slipped under the user to rest on top of the lavatory pan. It is filled with warm water from a jug (or by hose from a nearby tap) and empties straight into the lavatory through a plug-hole (Aremco);

2. A shower stool with a horse-shoe shaped seat may be a solution for those who need to wash or shower sitting down (Figure 5.16). It can be used in the shower stall, or standing in the bath in conjunction with a shower hose, but even by itself it provides a good well-supported position for an all over wash. There are many types of shower seats, some with arm and back supports, and some on wheels (Nottingham Rehab Ltd);

3. If the bath can be used there are hoists to assist in lifting the disabled person. There are special seats which can be fitted into the bath to make it easier to get in and out. A board fitted across the top of the bath makes it possible for someone who cannot stand to transfer from chair to bath. A shower hose bought

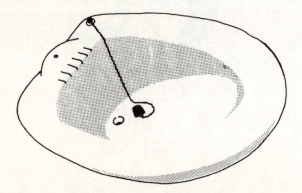

Figure 5.15   Portable bidet.

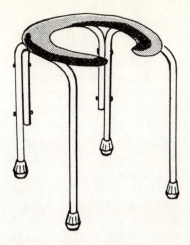

Figure 5.16   Shower stool with horse-shoe shaped seat.

from the chemist and fitted to the taps may make washing easier.

SUPPLY OF COMMODES AND OTHER AIDS

In many cases these are supplied through the social services department of the DHSS. Comprehensive descriptive lists, with details of manufacture and supply, and a guide to current prices, are kept by the Disabled Living Foundation, from whom information can be obtained. A wide variety of items is on permanent display at the DLF Equipment Centre in London.

CLOTHING

To someone who is incontinent, the choice of clothing is particularly important, as it can make the condition more manageable. Certain styles, easy fastenings and modern easy-care materials can facilitate this.

If there is a need to pass urine in a hurry, clothing which

is easy to remove or adjust quickly is essential. The following suggestions can be considered:

1. skirts and dresses should be neither too straight nor too full for easier management;
2. lined skirts eliminate the need for petticoats which only add another layer of clothing to be removed;
3. short vests and camisoles can be worn which do not have to be adjusted when passing urine:
4. camiknickers – these can be quickly pulled aside while passing urine;
5. for men, trousers with a full or partially elasticated waist are more quickly and easily managed; if an appliance is worn, a zip fastener in the inside seam of the trouser leg makes it easier to empty and change the bag (Figure 5.17);

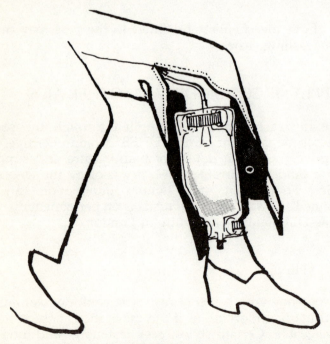

Figure 5.17 Trouser adaptation: zip fastener allows easy emptying and changing of the bag.

6. the wearing of underclothing like slips and boxer shorts allows for speed of action when the desire to pass water is felt;
7. as with bedlinen, clothing if wet or soiled should be rinsed and soaked immediately in cold water or Napisan (Boots Co. Ltd) to prevent odour and staining.

Physical disability

The clothing adviser at the Disabled Living Foundation will give advice about individual clothing and dressing problems where there are difficulties because of disability.

There are notes on clothing and dressing which can be purchased. Other useful publications are listed in Appendix C.

The Library
College of Nursing and Midwifery
City General Hospital
Stoke on Trent ST4 6QG

6
Protective equipment

In certain circumstances, urinary incontinence cannot be completely controlled. However, there are means of protection which help the wearer to be more comfortable and lead a normal life; these are collection devices and various forms of pads and pants.

Many types are available and choice depends on a number of different factors. If there is a continence nurse adviser in the area he or she will advise on what is suitable and available (see Appendix B). The following factors need to be considered:

1. how much urine is passed: does it leak out slowly or gush out; how often does the appliance bag or pad need to be changed?
2. pads can be used by either sex, but for men the pad needs to be shorter and placed in the front of the body; for women it should be placed centrally between the legs;
3. a different pad and pants system may be required for night time use, e.g. the Molnlycke system (see p. 53), whereas the Kanga pant system is only suitable for day time use.
4. check that the system is manageable if there is difficulty in standing or difficulty with hand movements;
5. are there suitable washing facilities or a means of disposing of pads?

COLLECTION DEVICES

These include penile sheaths, bodyworn appliances, dribble pouches, and a variety of pads and pants.

Penile sheath

This is a condom sheath which fits over the penis, and is attached to a bag by a tube (Figure 6.1). The sheath can be

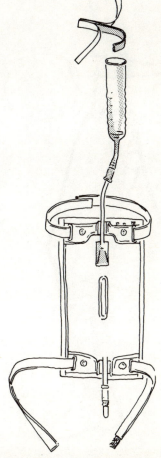

Figure 6.1 Condom sheath.

held in place by an adhesive strip which adheres to the
penis on one side and to the sheath on the other. Spray-on
adhesives are also available. The sheath should be sized to
slip easily over the penis allowing for any size change in
the penis. There are firms which supply an initial sizing
pack (Coloplast Ltd; Aldington Laboratories Ltd). The
penile sheath system is suitable for moderate to severe
incontinence.

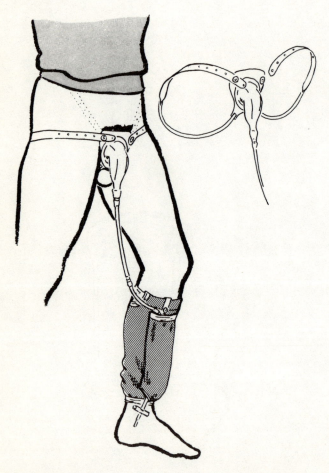

Figure 6.2 Bodyworn urinal and calf bag holder.

Bodyworn appliances

Many bodyworn appliances are available, and it is essential to seek the advice of a skilled fitter. These appliances fit over the penis, and some enclose the scrotum. Urine is collected in a bag which can be attached to the leg and concealed inside the trouser leg (Figure 6.2). (Simcare; Payne; Thackraycare Ltd; Bard Ltd).

There are specially designed thigh and calf garments for holding the bag which are comfortable to wear (Figure 6.3). (Squibb Surgicare Ltd; Brevet Hospital Products Ltd).

The important points are that the appliance fits, that it has a suitable capacity for the type of incontinence and that it is easy for the person to put on and take off. Since it needs to be washed and dried regularly, two appliances

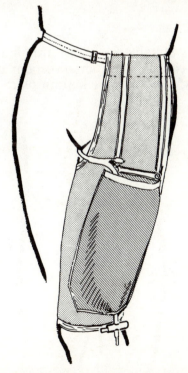

Figure 6.3 Bag holder for female wearing a catheter.

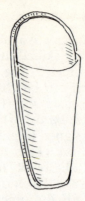

Figure 6.4 Dribble pouch.

are needed, although the first should be tried out before a second is purchased.

Dribble pouches

These are only suitable for slight dribbling incontinence. The pouches consist of super-absorbent material with a plastic backing which can be kept in place by mesh pants

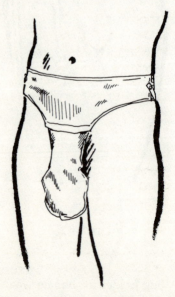

Figure 6.5 Washable dribble pouch.

or other close-fitting pants (Figure 6.4) (Coloplast Ltd; LIC Ltd).

A washable dribble pouch attached to a waistband is available. This can be filled with cotton wool or wadding and changed as necessary (Figure 6.5) (Simcare).

Pads and pants

There are no satisfactory appliances for women to wear. The use of absorbent pads and protective pants are an alternative solution. Many are available but there are four basic types:

1. plastic pants into which pads are placed. There are pull-on, drop-front, and side-opening styles. The pants are waterproof but tend to be hot and sticky and the plastic becomes hardened. Skin damage may result from excessive sweating (Henleys Medical Supplies Ltd);
2. the Marsupial Pants (Kanga, Nicholas Laboratories Ltd) or similar garment (Hygicare Ltd; Ganmill Ltd; Boots Co. Ltd) were designed to keep the urine and plastic away from the skin (Figure. 6.6).

   Marsupial Pants are made of knitted one-way fabric through which the urine passes to be absorbed by a pad which is held in a plastic pouch on the *outside* of the garment. Provided the pad is changed regularly, the pants and the body of the wearer remain dry. The pad can be changed without removing the pants, although it is necessary to raise the body slightly to do this. A close fit is necessary and sizing is by hip measurement. There are both pull-on and open-flat drop-front styles. They are not suitable for night wear or for double incontinence.

   Styles include side-opening and drop-front with velcro fastenings which allow for easy changing; Kanga Lady, made of floral material, is neat but the pad holds less urine; the Y-front style for men allows both for normal urination and protection. Special pads are supplied with all of these;
3. pants made of stretch nylon mesh which hold in place a plastic-backed pad are also available (Figure

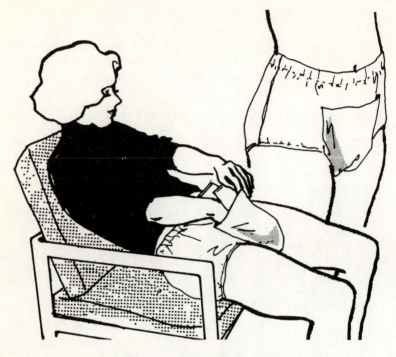

Figure 6.6   Kanga type pants.

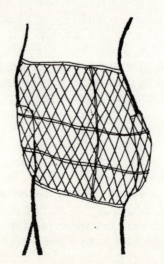

Figure 6.7   Mesh pants.

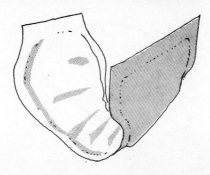

Figure 6.8 Tenaform shaped pad.

6.7). They stretch to fit wearers of any size, and are extremely light and comfortable. A large size is available.

The plastic-backed shaped pads (Figure 6.8) to be worn with these vary in size. They range from one dealing with light incontinence to one for heavy and night incontinence (Tenaform, Molnlycke Ltd). Other plastic-backed pads are oblong in shape (Robinsons; Vernon Carus Ltd).

4. The fourth type is a completely disposable all-in-one pant and pad (Figure 6.9). It looks like, and is based on, the disposable baby nappy. Although the appearance may be off-putting, it is effective protection for heavy incontinence (Caducee Health Care; Ancilla; Molnlycke Ltd).

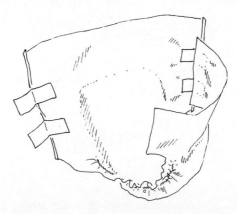

Figure 6.9 Disposable pad and pants.

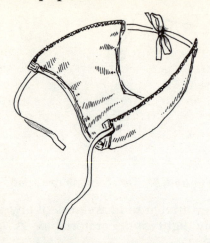

Figure 6.10 Washable pad.

Other pads

Some pads are washable and therefore re-usable (Figure 6.10). They are made of spun polyester with waterproof backing and are kept in place by tapes and used under stretch pants or normal underwear (Ganmill Ltd).

There are also pants with a built-in special fabric in the crotch which absorbs the urine (Figure 6.11). The pants are washed in the normal way. These are suitable for light incontinence, e.g. stress incontinence (Ganmill Ltd; Nicholas Laboratories Ltd).

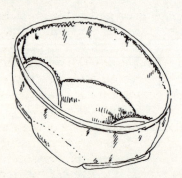

Figure 6.11 Washable pants with absorbent fabric.

BED PROTECTION

Bedpads are an underpad consisting of a paper surface, wadding and a plastic back. They can be placed across the bed, but are often inadequate if large amounts of urine are passed, although there are two types which are thicker and better than the others (Smith & Nephew Ltd; Ancilla). If an underpad is used it should be placed across the bed under the buttocks, not lengthwise. The larger size is more appropriate (75 × 57 cm; 30 × 23 in).

The Kylie drawsheet is washable and tucks into each side of the bed. It is made of a quilted absorbent material, which soaks up the urine, spreads it and keeps the body comparatively dry (Nicholas Laboratories Ltd). There are also other smaller, washable sheets made of different absorbent materials (ACS Medical; Gimson Tendercare).

ODOUR

If odour is a problem there are neutralizing deodorants. One example, Nilodor, is effective if a drop or two is placed on protective padding, or into any appliance or urinal (Loxley Medical, Boots Co. Ltd).

PERSONAL CARE

The skin should be kept as dry as possible by frequent changing of underpads or pads. If urine is left on the skin or clothing, it decomposes and ammonia (an alkali) is released which irritates the skin and produces a smell.

Wash the area with a soft cloth and ordinary soap and water before renewing the pad. A barrier cream can prevent soreness. If talcum powder is used, use it sparingly. Washing may be difficult, especially if there is any disability; a tissue or cloth covering a foam mop may help. Sometimes special wet-sealed medical tissues are helpful. A portable bidet may be useful for someone able to use the lavatory (see p. 42) as it can be placed on top of the lavatory for washing purposes.

LAUNDRY

If linen is soiled it should be rinsed out and soaked in cold water in a covered bucket. Napisan can be added to help the cleaning action. The article can then be washed in the normal way and no staining or smell should result. Biological washing powders are sometimes used, but care should be taken as these are strong and may irritate the skin. A special laundry service may be available in the area; enquire about this (see Chapter 7).

Used disposable pads should be put in a plastic bag inside another closed container. In this way any smell which may arise from decomposing excreta is avoided.

7
Services available

There are a number of services to help those who are incontinent. Unfortunately embarrassment sometimes prevents people from asking and finding out what can be done. The following is a guide to available services, though resources vary widely from one area to another.

HEALTH SERVICES

Doctor

The family doctor will supply the initial medical advice, and arrange for a visit to a specialist or specialized hospital centre if necessary (incontinence/urodynamic clinic).

District (home) nurse

If nursing advice and assistance are required, the doctor will arrange for the district nurse to call. In some areas a nursing auxiliary may assist with daily bathing and dressing, and night nursing can sometimes be arranged for those patients who may require it. The district nurse, as a member of the primary health care team, will maintain continuity of care, when necessary, between hospital and home.

Continence nurse adviser

The continence nurse adviser, if available, may be referred to for incontinence problems.

Health visitor

The health visitor is a nurse with additional training to enable him or her to advise on a number of points including health education and social needs. He or she can fulfil these functions when visiting disabled or elderly people in their own home, and will attempt to sort out what kind of help should be given in consultation with the patient, the family, and, if necessary, with other members of the care team including the social worker.

Practical help available

The district nurse, health visitor or continence nurse adviser can advise about the following:

1. the supply and use of equipment such as urinals, protective pants, pads, bedpads, etc;
2. incontinent laundry service to collect soiled linen and sometimes nightclothes;
3. disposal service to collect soiled pads and bedpads. There may be a special collection, or bags may be supplied to put out with ordinary refuse. This service is usually run by the Cleansing Department of the Council.

SOCIAL SERVICES

Social worker

The social worker from the Social Services Department of the Local Authority can help with individual or family stress, and advise about practical help available. In many areas there are also occupational therapists who can give practical advice. The following services may be available:

1. home help: to help with housework, sometimes with laundry, and sometimes with personal needs such as washing, dressing, shopping or collecting pension;
2. laundry service: see also previous mention under

Health Services. This is run by the Social Services
Department in some areas;

3. the Social Services Department will advise about
   alterations and adaptations to the home which may
   make it easier for a disabled person to manage – for
   instance if the bathroom or lavatory is inaccessible. If
   the house belongs to the Council this will be done in
   consultation with the Housing Department. The Social Services Department will advise and help about
   alterations to privately owned or rented houses;

4. it may be possible for a holiday to be arranged for the
   incontinent person. RADAR issues an annual guide
   Holidays for the Physically Handicapped, in which details are given of holiday accommodation where
   incontinent guests are accepted. Some organizations
   also run their own holiday homes as well as a
   Holiday Care Service. The social worker can advise
   and help with arrangements;

5. equipment such as commodes, chemical closets and
   special chairs can also be supplied. The Red Cross
   and other voluntary organizations may lend equipment at short notice for a temporary period.

The address of the Social Services Department can be
obtained from the local Town Hall or Post Office, or from
the doctor or nurse, or can be found in the telephone
directory.

FINANCIAL HELP

Attendance Allowance: this is a tax-free allowance for
those who require a considerable amount of care during
the day or night, or both. It is paid to disabled people, but
those with problems of incontinence will be considered.

Income Support – Provision for Exceptional Needs: for
anyone already receiving income support or pension there
may be an additional allowance payable for extra expenses
incurred, such as those on heating and laundry. Enquiries
about financial aid should be made at the local Social
Security Office, the address of which can be obtained from

the Post Office. For those unable to call at their local office, a visit at home can be requested.

Appendix A

Suppliers of protective equipment and aids to continence.

ACS Medical	Kestrel House, Garth Road, Morden, Surrey SM4 4LP (tel. 01 330 4333)
Aldington Laboratories Ltd	Mersham, Ashford, Kent (tel. 023372 482)
Ancilla	*see* **Molnlyke Ltd**
Aremco	Grove House, Lenham, Kent ME17 2PX
Bard C. R. Ltd	Bard Urology Division, Pennywell Industrial Estate, Sunderland, Co. Durham, Tyne and Wear SR4 9EW (tel. 091 534 3131)
John Bell and Croydon Ltd	50–54 Wigmore Street, London W1H 0AU (tel. 01 935 5555)
Boots Co. Ltd	(large branches)
Brevet Hospital Products Ltd	Unit 1–3 Weymills, Whitchurch, Shropshire SY13 1N (tel. 0948 4487)
Caducee Health Care	Rye Park Industrial Estate, Rye Road, Hoddesdon, Herts EN11 0EL (tel. 0992 445658)

Coloplast Ltd	Peterborough Business Park, Peterborough, Cambs PE2 0FX (tel. 0733 239898)
Franklin Medical Ltd	PO Box 138, Cressex Industrial Estate, High Wycombe, Bucks HP12 3NB (tel. 0494 32761)
Freeman William and Co. Ltd	Suba-Seal Works, Wakefield Road, Staincross, Barnsley, S. Yorks S75 6DH (tel. 0226 24081)
Ganmill Ltd	38–40 Market Street, Bridgewater, Somerset TA6 3EP (tel. 0278 423037)
Gimson Tendercare	62 Boston Road, Beaumont Leys, Leicester LE14 1AZ (tel. 0533 366779)
Henleys Medical Supplies Ltd	Alexandra Works, Clarendon Road, London N8 0DL (tel. 01 889 3151)
Hygicare Ltd	1 Macon Court, Macon Way, Crewe, Cheshire CW1 1EA (tel. 0270 580061)
LIC Ltd	129 Grovley Road, Sunbury-on-Thames, Middx TW16 7JZ (tel. 01 751 1141)
Loxley Medical	Unit 5D Carnaby Industrial Estate, Bridlington YO15 3QY (tel. 0262 603979)
Molnlycke Ltd	Southfields Road, Dunstable, Beds LU6 3EJ (tel. 0582 600211)
Nicholas Laboratories Ltd	225 Bath Road, Slough SL1 4AU (tel. 0753 23971)
Nicholls & Clarke Ltd	Niclar House, 3–10 Shoreditch High Street, London E1 6PE (tel. 01 247 5432)

The Library
College of Nursing and Midwifery
City General Hospital
Stoke on Trent ST4 6QG

Nottingham Rehab Ltd	17 Ludlow Hill Road, Melton Road, West Bridgford, Nottingham, Notts NG2 6HD (tel. 0602 234251)
Payne S. G. & P.	81 Hollins Lane, Marple Bridge, Cheshire SK6 5DA (tel. 061 427 7423)
Robinsons of Chesterfield	Wheat Bridge, Chesterfield, Derbyshire S40 2AD (tel. 0482 25181)
Simcare Eshman Bros & Walsh Ltd	Peter Road, Lancing, West Sussex BN15 8TJ (tel. 0903 761122)
Smith & Nephew Ltd	81 Hessle Road, Hull HU3 2BN (tel. 0482 25181)
Squibb Surgicare Ltd	141–9 Staines Road, Hounslow, Middx TW3 3JA (tel. 01 572 7422)
Thackraycare Ltd	47 Great George Street, Leeds LS1 3BB (tel. 0532 430028)
Vernon Carus Ltd	Penwortham Mills, Preston PR1 9SN (tel. 0772 744493)

Appendix B

Useful addresses

Association of Continence Advisers	c/o The Disabled Living Foundation, 380–4 Harrow Road, London W9 2HU (tel. 01 289 6111)
Association for Spina Bifida and Hydrocephalus	22 Upper Woburn Place, London WC1H 0EP (tel. 01 388 1382)
British Epilepsy Association	Anstey House, 40 Hanover Square, Leeds LS3 1BE (tel. 0532 439393)
British Red Cross Society	9 Grosvenor Crescent, London SW1X 7EJ (tel. 01 235 5454)
Chest, Heart and Stroke Association	Tavistock House North, Tavistock Square, London WC1H 9JE (tel. 01 387 3012)
Colostomy Welfare Group	38–9 Eccleston Square, London SW1V 1PD (tel. 01 828 5175)
Disabled Living Foundation	Incontinence Advisory Service, 380–4 Harrow Road, London W9 2HU (tel. 01 289 6111)

Disablement Income Group (DIG)	Millmead Business Centre, Millmead Road, London N17 9QU (tel. 01 801 8013)
Ileostomy Association of Great Britain and Ireland (IA)	Amblehurst House, Black Scotch Lane, Mansfield, Notts NG18 4PF (tel. 0623 28099)
International Continence Society	Mr Paul Abrams, Dept of Urology, Southmead Hospital, Bristol BS10 5NB
Invalid Children's Aid Association (ICAA)	1st Floor, Herald House, Lamb's Passage, London EC1 8LE (tel. 01 628 2185 or 01 375 0247)
Multiple Sclerosis Society of Great Britain & Northern Ireland	25 Effie Road, London SW6 1EE (tel. 01 381 4022)
Muscular Dystrophy Group of Great Britain	Natrass House, 35 Macaulay Road, London SW4 0QP (tel. 01 720 8055)
MENCAP	Mencap National Centre, 123 Golden Lane, London EC1Y 0RT (tel. 01 253 9433)
RADAR (Royal Association Disability and Rehabilitation)	25 Mortimer Street, London W1N 8AB (tel. 01 637 5400)
Spastics Society	12 Park Crescent, London W1N 4EQ (tel. 01 636 5020)
Spinal Injuries Association	New Point House, 76 St James's Lane, London N10 3DF (tel. 01 444 2121)
SPOD (Sexual and Personal Relationships of the Disabled)	286 Camden Road, London N7 0BJ (tel. 01 607 8851)

DISABLED LIVING CENTRES OFFERING A COMPREHENSIVE SERVICE

The Disabled Living Centres listed below are centres where a selection of aids for disabled people can be seen and tried out. They have been set up to provide information to those professionally concerned with disability and to disabled people and their friends and relations. As the Centres vary considerably in size, content and the kind of services they offer, it is wise to check that the purpose of the visit can be fulfilled.

Visitors should always contact the centre before visiting as an appointment is usually necessary.

Belfast	**Disabled Living Centre**, Prosthetic Orthotic and Aids Service, Musgrave Park Hospital, Stockman's Lane, Belfast BT9 7JB (tel. 0232 669501)
Birmingham	**Disabled Living Centre**, 260 Broad Street, Birmingham B1 2HF (tel. 021 643 0980)
Caerphilly	**Resources (Aids and Equipment) Centre**, Wales Council for the Disabled, Caerbragdy Industrial Estate, Bedwas Road, Caerphilly, Mid Glamorgan CF8 3SL (tel. 0222 887325 or 887326/7)
Cardiff	**The Demonstration Aids Centre**, The Lodge, Rookwood Hospital, Llandaff, Cardiff, South Glamorgan CF5 2YN (tel. 0222 566281 x 5166)
Edinburgh	**Disabled Living Centre**, Astley Ainslie Hospital, Grange Loan, Edinburgh EH9 2HL (tel. 031 447 6271 x 5653)
Leeds	**The William Merritt Disabled Living Centre**, St Mary's Hospital, Greenhill Rd, Leeds LS12 3QE (tel. 0532 793140)
Leicester	**T.R.A.I.D.S.** (Trent Region Aids, Information and Demonstration Service), 76 Clarendon Park Road, Leicester LE2 3AD (tel. 0533 700747 or 7008748)

Liverpool	**Merseyside Centre for Independent Living**, Youens Way, East Prescott Road, Liverpool LE14 2EP (tel. 051 228 9221)
London	**Disabled Living Foundation Equipment Centre**, 380–4 Harrow Road, London W9 2HU (tel. 01 289 6111)
Manchester	**Disabled Living Services**, Disabled Living Centre, Redbank House, 4 St Chad's Street, Cheetham, Manchester M8 8QA (tel. 061 832 3678)
Newcastle upon Tyne	**Newcastle upon Tyne Council for the Disabled**, The Dene Centre, Castles Farm Road, Newcastle upon Tyne NE3 1PH (tel. 091 284 0480)
Nottingham	**Nottingham Resource Centre for the Disabled**, Lenton Business Centre, Lenton Boulevard, Nottingham NG7 2BY (tel. 0602 420391)
Sheffield	**Sheffield Independent Living Centre**, 108 The Moor, Sheffield S1 4DP (tel. 0742 737025)
Southampton	**Southampton Aid and Equipment Centre**, Southampton General Hospital, Tremona Road, Southampton SO9 4XY (tel. 0703 777222 x 3414 or 3233)
Stockport	**Disabled Living Centre**, Stockport Area Health Authority, St Thomas's Hospital, Shawhead, Stockport SK3 8BL (tel. 061 419 4476)
Swindon	**The Swindon Centre for Disabled Living**, The Hawthorn Centre, Cricklade Road, Swindon, Wilts SN2 1AF (tel. 0793 643966)

MOBILE ADVICE CENTRE

Scottish Council on Disability	Princes House, 5 Shandwick Place, Edinburgh EH2 4RG (tel. 031 229 8632)

(This is a travelling exhibition which tours Scotland. Contact the organization for details of the places to be visited. Appointments are not necessary.)

OTHER PLACES WHERE AIDS AND EQUIPMENT MAY BE SEEN (please ring for appointment)

Local occupational therapy departments in hospitals; local social services departments (some have assessment centres).

The Spastics Society   16 Fitzroy Square, London W1P 5HQ (tel. 01 387 9571) (have an assessment centre for children).

As new Disabled Living Centres are planned contact: **Disabled Living Centres Council, c/o TRAIDS** (Trent Region Aids, Information and Demonstration Service), 76 Clarendon Park Road, Leicester LE2 3AD (tel. 0533 700747/8) for details of proposed new centres in other parts of the country.

Appendix C

Further reading

BOOKS FOR THE GENERAL PUBLIC

Feneley, R. C. L. and Blannin, J. P. (1984) *Incontinence*, Patient handbook series 18, Churchill Livingstone, Edinburgh.
Meadow, R. (1980) *Help for Bedwetting*, Churchill Livingstone, Edinburgh.
(Useful for mothers, children and adults. A short practical guide)
Montgomery, E. (1974) *Regaining Bladder Control*, John Wright, Bristol.
(Detailed instructions in pelvic floor re-education)
Turnbull, P. and Ruston, R. (1985) *Clothes Sense For Disabled People of all Ages*, rev. edn. London, Disabled Living Foundation.

BOOKS FOR FURTHER READING

Association of Continence Advisers (1988) *Directory of Continence Aids and Appliances*, 4th edn ACA, London.
(Reference book for nurses and other professionals)
Browne, B. (1978) *Management for Continence*. Mitcham, Age Concern England.
(A useful guide for those working in residential accommodation)
Department of Health and Social Security (1986) *Incontinence Garments: Results of a DHSS study* Health Equipment Information, no 159. DHSS Scientific and Technical Branch, STBI, Room 213, 14 Russell Square, London WC1B 5EP.

Mandelstam, D. (ed.) (1986) *Incontinence and its Management*, 2nd edn Croom Helm, London.
(A text book with contributions from doctors, nurses and others on aspects of management)
Mandelstam, D. and Lane, P. (1981). *Incontinence Bibliography* Disabled Living Foundation, London.
Norton, C. (1986) *Nursing for Continence*, Beaconsfield Publishers, Beaconsfield.
(Textbook on nursing management)

DISABLED LIVING FOUNDATION INCONTINENCE ADVISORY SERVICE LEAFLETS

Adult Bedwetting (nocturnal enuresis): causes, sources of help; suggested remedies.

Bedwetting (nocturnal enuresis): extract from *Notes on Childhood Incontinence* on causes, sources of help.

Bladder Training: information on self-help for people with certain types of bladder problems.

Confused Incontinent Person at Home: general help and information.

Faecal Incontinence: set of notes for professionals.

Management of Bowels: checklist and guidelines for professionals.

Notes on Childhood Incontinence: general notes for professionals and public.

Notes on Incontinence: general notes for professionals and public.

Penile Sheaths: general notes for professionals and public.

Stress Incontinence: extract from *Notes on Incontinence*, includes pelvic floor exercises.

Urinary Incontinence: checklist and guidelines for professionals.

Washable Bed Protection: general guidelines for professionals and public.

Your Prostate Operation: general notes for professionals and public.

DLF CLOTHING ADVISORY SERVICE LEAFLETS

CC1 *Clothing for continence – women* (Sept 1987).
CC2 *Clothing for continence – men* (Sept 1987).

CC3 *Clothing for men who are incontinent* (Sept 1987).
CC4 *Clothing for women who are incontinent* (Sept 1987).

DLF INFORMATION SERVICE DISABILITY EQUIPMENT HANDBOOK SECTIONS

Section 1A *Beds & bed accessories.*
Section 7A *Personal toilet.*

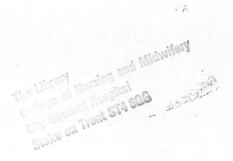

The Library
College of Nursing and Midwifery
City General Hospital
Stoke on Trent ST4 6QG

Glossary

Alimentary canal	the whole channel through which food passes from the mouth to the anus.
Anus	back passage. A ring-like opening at the end of the bowel through which solid faeces are finally passed.
Artery	muscular tube conveying blood from the heart to all parts of the body.
Bladder	a bag-like structure in which urine is collected. It lies in the pelvis in front of the bowels.
Bowels	also called intestines. The alimentary canal below the stomach through which food travels to the anus. It is 33 ft (10 m) long in the average adult.
Catheter	a thin flexible tube introduced into the bladder to withdraw urine.
Coma	deep unconsciousness.
Congenital	dating from birth.
Continence	the ability to control bladder and bowel functions.
Cystitis	infection of the bladder.
Detrusor	the emptying muscle of the bladder.
Diuretic	a substance such as a drug which stimulates the kidneys to produce urine (water pills).
Double incontinence	a condition where both urinary and faecal incontinence exist.

Dribbling   a flow of urine in drops or a trickling stream.

Enuresis   bedwetting usually applied to children, but can also apply to adults.

Excreta   waste expelled from the body, i.e. urine and faeces.

Faeces   waste matter emptied from the bowel; sometimes called a motion or stool

Fibroids   benign growths in the womb.

Gynaecology   the study of disease in women, especially of the reproductive system.

Geriatric medicine   the study of the health and welfare of old people.

Infection   disease-producing germs on or in the body.

Intestines (see bowels)   bowels from stomach to anus.

Lax   loose, relaxed.

Micturition   urination, passing water.

Overflow incontinence   dribbling urine from an over-full bladder.

Pelvis   bony basin at lower end of the spine.

Pelvic floor   two flat sheets of muscle which approximate in the mid line, and through which the urethra, the vagina (female) and the bowel pass.

Penis   the male organ through which the urethra passes.

Polyuria   the production of large quantities of urine.

Precipitancy   the passing of urine with awareness but no warning.

Prolapse   the slipping forward or downward of part of an organ such as the womb or rectum.

Prostate   a gland in men which lies below the bladder and surrounds the upper part of the urethra.

Rectum	the final part of the bowel which terminates in the anus.
Reflex	an automatic response.
Scrotum	bag containing the testicles.
Sign	evidence of disease which the doctor observes.
Symptom	that which the patient is aware of.
Spinal cord	a rope-like mass of nerve cells and fibres which can transmit messages from the brain and the tissues of the body.
Sphincter	ring of muscle guarding or closing an opening in the body, i.e. anal sphincter.
Stoma	small mouth-like opening made artificially from a hollow organ like the bowel or bladder to the skin surface.
Stress incontinence	a small leakage of urine which occurs on any unusual exertion such as coughing, laughing or sneezing.
Stroke	paralysis arising from brain damage.
Trauma	injury.
Trigone	triangular shaped base of the bladder.
Ureters	two tubes which convey urine from the kidneys to the bladder.
Urethra	the outlet tube from the bladder. 1½ in (3.75 cm) long in the female, and 6–8 in (15–20 cm) in the male.
Urgency	a pressing and urgent desire to pass water.
Urine	fluid from the kidneys stored in the bladder and voided through the urethra at intervals.
Urinate	to pass urine.
Urinary diversion	a method of emptying urine through an artificial opening made in the wall of the abdomen, or by transplanting the ureters into the wall of the bowel.
Urinary retention	inability to pass urine, and consequent over-filling of the bladder.

Urology   the study of diseases of the urinary system.

Uterus   womb. The female organ within which the child is conceived, situated between the bladder and the rectum.

Uterine   connected with the uterus.

Vagina   front passage in the female leading to the uterus.

Womb   see uterus.

Index

Aids to continence, suppliers
    61–3, 68
Arthritis and urinary
    incontinence 12
Association of Continence
    Advisers ix
Associations 64–8
Attendance allowance 59

Bathing aids 42
Bed protection 55
Bedwetting 2
    adult 7
    treatment 25
Bidet, portable 42
Bladder
    anatomy 5
    control 7
    leakage, types 9
    training, in urge
        incontinence 21
Bodyworn appliances 49
Bowel action, natural
    variations 14
    anatomy 15
    control 28
    incontinence 14–17

Catheterization, intermittent
    28

long-term 23
sexual intercourse during
    24, 65
Children, incontinence 2
Closets, chemical 37
Clothing Advisory Service
    leaflets (DLF) 70
Clothing 43
Collection devices 47
Commodes 36, 43
Condom as collection device
    47
Continence Advisers,
    Association of ix
Continence
    aids 31–45
    nurse adviser 57
Cushions, cut out 37

Defaecation, natural
    variations 14
Deodorants 55
Diuretics 13
Disseminated (multiple)
    sclerosis and
    incontinence 29
Dribble pouches 50

Emotional factors in urinary
    incontinence 11

78 Index

Enuresis, nocturnal 7, 9
management 25
Exercises in treatment of stress
incontinence 20

Faecal incontinence 14–17
causes 16
persistent 17
prevention 16
Financial help 59
Frequency, management 21
Freud on excretion 3

Glossary 72–5

Hospitalization and
incontinence 29

Income support 59
Incontinence
Advisory Service ix
leaflets (DLF) 70
definition of 1
double 16
emotional factors 11
faecal 14–17
causes 16
persistent 17
prevention 16
in hospital 29
personal care 55
urinary incontinence 5–13
causes 9
due to physical
disabilities 22
history of treatment 2
management 18–30
catheterization 23
in stroke 28

nocturnal 7,9,11
overflow 9–10
management 22
reflex 9, 11
stress 9
management 19, 23
urge 9, 10

Kanga pants 51

Laundry 51
Lavatory, aids in 38–41

Marsupial pants 51
Medicines as cause of
incontinence 13
Mesh pants 51
Multiple sclerosis and
incontinence 29

Overflow incontinence,
management 22

Pads 46, 51–4
washable 54
Pants 46, 51–4
Personal care in incontinence
55
Physical difficulties in urge
incontinence 22
Prostate, enlarged, and
overflow incontinence 22
Protective equipment 45–56
suppliers 61–3

St Peter's boat 33
Services available for
incontinent people 57–60

Sexual intercourse and
   incontinence 24, 65
Shower stool 43
Social services for incontinent
   people 58
Spinal injury and bladder
   control 27, 28
Stress incontinence 9
   management 19, 23
Stroke, incontinence in 26
Suba–Seal urinal 33
Suppliers of protective
   equipment 61–3
Surgery in stress incontinence
   21

Treatment of incontinence 2,
   18–30
Urge incontinence,
   management 21
Urinals, bodyworn 48, 49
   female 33
   male 31
   swan-type 33
Urinary tract, surgical
   diversion 27
Urine, collection devices 47

Walking frames, lavatory use
   41
Washing aids 42